Arterial Blood Gas Interpretation
by
Jamie Bisson

(Dip H.Sc., Dip. N.Sc., BSc. (Hons.)
Crit. Care)

Foreword

I am a clinical nurse specialist working in a major tertiary referral centre within Australia. I qualified in 1998 and since then I have been working in critical care, more specifically in a coronary care unit, cardiac high dependency units, cardiothoracic intensive care units, a paediatric and a general intensive care unit. In addition to this I have worked as an educator in all of my places of work.

I believe that arterial blood gas (ABG) analysis is a relatively simple task which can be taught to anyone given the right instruction and information. Whether you are studying for an assignment, working in critical care, or just wanting to further your knowledge then this simple book will teach you exactly what you need to know in an easy to understand step by step process.

In addition to this resource, more resources are available from our website:

http://www.eadvancedhealthcare.com/healthcare-resources/

Table Of Contents

Introduction

ABG's are done routinely in caring for critically ill patients and their evaluation is crucial for the safe and effective care of the patient[1]. ABGs can be broken down into several subsections including oxygenation, metabolic parameters and acid base balance. This book is designed to provide you with the necessary steps and information necessary to make an informed decision with regard to the treatment of the patient.

What Is An Arterial Blood Gas?

An ABG is a sample of blood taken from an artery. The blood sample is tested for several dissolved substances and gasses, substances like potassium, sodium, haemoglobin, sodium bicarbonate, calcium, glucose and lactate. The gases examined include oxygen and carbon dioxide.

The sample can be taken from any artery, however it is mainly taken from the radial artery in the wrist, or the brachial artery on the back of the elbow, or the femoral artery in the crease of the groin[2], as shown next:

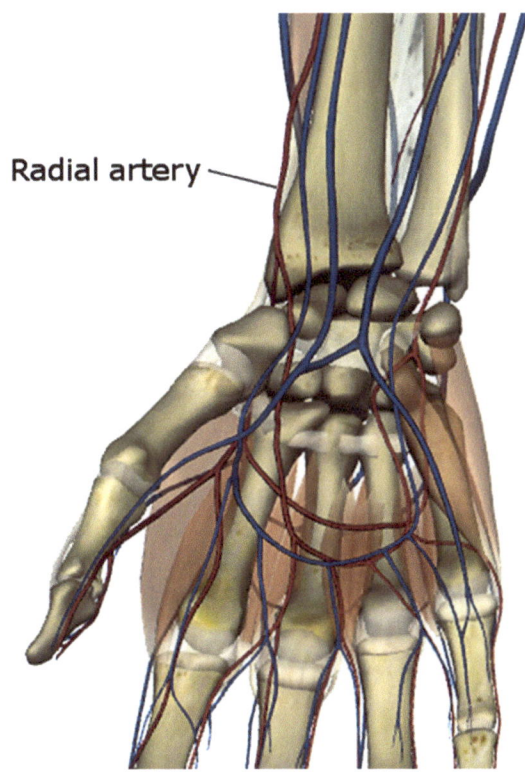

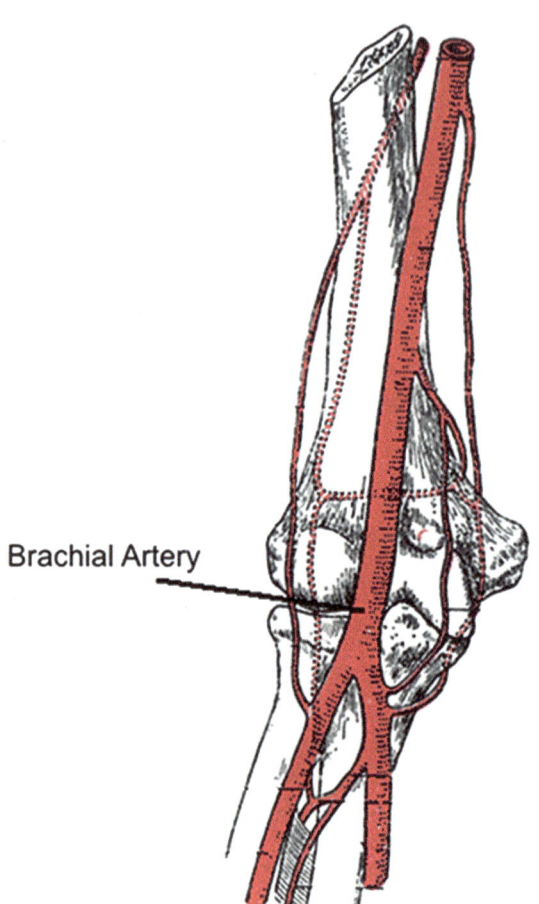

Brachial Artery

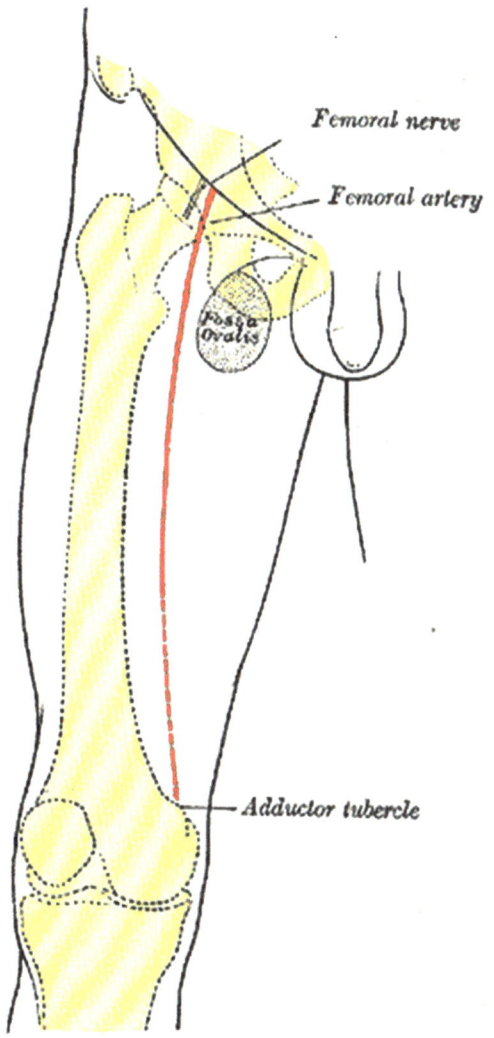

Femoral nerve

Femoral artery

Fossa Ovalis

Adductor tubercle

Once the sample has been taken all the air should be expelled from the syringe and a cap placed on the top of the syringe to reduce the risk of further gaseous exchange within the sample from the outside air. Ideally the sample should be analysed immediately, however if this is not possible it should be analysed within 30 minutes and kept at room temperature[3]. The sample should also be agitated before analysis to ensure that there is a well mixed sample available to the blood gas machine. The mixing of the blood sample in the syringe is also important as it freely mixes the dry heparin within the syringe, which reduces the risk of clots forming in the machine. Often after a while, coagulation occurs at the top of the syringe, so ideally a few drops of blood should be expelled from the syringe before sampling. The coagulation, in practice, only occurs after a prolonged period and is not an issue when the sample is analysed immediately.

How To Take The Sample

There are 2 main ways of taking an arterial blood gas, namely with an arterial puncture or through an arterial line. Both methods have their advantages and disadvantages: With an arterial puncture the patient will feel some discomfort; it may also be difficult to locate the artery especially when the patient is shocked or critically unwell such as in an emergency; there is also a risk of nerve injury with attempting to puncture the artery as the nerves run extremely nearby[3]. There is also a risk of needle-stick injury with taking an arterial blood gas with the arterial puncture method[3]. An arterial line however, takes some time and skill to insert and has an inherent risk of infection for the patient, there is also an increased risk of a thrombus in the artery; and air embolus is another risk with an arterial line[3]. There is also the risk that the arterial line may become disconnected and the patient would then lose a significant amount of blood should the issue not be identified swiftly[3].

In additions to the 2 main methods of taking an arterial blood gas, as mentioned previously, capillary blood gas sampling is also possible and is often used with paediatrics and neonates. Again this method has its own problems: the skills needed to collect the sample are significant; the child will also experience a fair amount of discomfort during the procedure; entraining air in the sample is also a concern; finally there is also an increased risk of the sample coagulating before being analysed.

What do all the Arterial Blood Gas Values Mean?

pH

pH is a scientific term which refers to the acidity or alkalinity of a substance. The scale of pH ranges from 1 to 14. The lower the pH, the more acidic a substance is. Inversely, the higher the pH the more alkaline the substance is. For example a pH of 1 is very acidotic and a pH of 14 is very alkalotic. The pH is a relative figure based on the concentration of hydrogen ions in the blood. Hydrogen ions are acidic and therefore an abundance of these causes acidosis.

Human blood has a very fine normal level, which is between 7.35 and 7.45[2]. This is balanced with many substances, which will be discussed later. A pH of less than 7.0 has a very high mortality rate[4].

The pH of a sample is affected by several factors, which will be discussed later.

PaO$_2$

"Pa" stands for the partial pressure of a gas dissolved in the artery. O$_2$ is obviously oxygen, a gas which is essential for cell respiration and activity. A normal PaO$_2$ is anywhere between 83 - 108mmHg or 11.1 - 14.4kPa[3]. If the PaO$_2$ is too low then the hypoxaemia will occur and there will be the potential for cell ischaemia, necrosis and death.

It is one of the main aims of every clinician to ensure that the patient is adequately oxygenated. Oxygenation at the cellular level is dependent upon the amount of oxygen inspired, the adequacy of gas transport through the alveoli, the affinity of oxygen to bind to haemoglobin, cardiac function, pulmonary circulation, systemic circulation and oxygen release.

We as clinicians give oxygen to our patients to alleviate the issue of hypoxia secondary to a low inspired oxygen concentration. The adequacy of gas transport through the alveoli is affected by a collapse in the patient's lungs, which is often alleviated by chest drains or an increase in the level of PEEP (positive and expiratory pressure), either on a ventilator or non-invasively with the use of BiPAP or CPAP. In some circumstances the patient may be in pulmonary oedema and frusemide may be indicated. The patient may also have an empyema or chest infection, which will affect gas transportation through the alveoli. In hyperthermia and acidaemia there is a decrease in the affinity that oxygen has to haemoglobin and as such oxygen will struggle to bind to haemoglobin[5]. Inversely in this state, oxygen will release from haemoglobin to the cells easily[5]. Understandably therefore in hypothermia and alkalosis oxygen has an increased affinity to haemoglobin and will bind easily to it, however when it needs to release at the cellular level it is more difficult[5]. This concept will be discussed later, but the understanding is based around shifts to the left and the right of the oxygen dissociation curve.

Cardiac function can be assessed using a multitude of skills, however one way of assessing cardiac function is to take a venous blood gas sample from the central line. If the PaO_2 is satisfactory and the $ScvO_2$ is lower than 70 then that may be indicative of a decreased cardiac function[6]. This test however would not be diagnostic in itself, but would give weight to a diagnosis of decreased cardiac function in the background of other clinical observations being made[7]. Inotropes, fluids or other medications may be necessary to improve cardiac function. Pulmonary and systemic circulation may also need to be supported with fluids, vasopressors, inotropes or broncho/vasodilators. Oxygen release at the cellular level is affected by temperature, pH and the presence of 2-3 DPG. 2 - 3 DPG will be discussed later.

PaCO$_2$

CO$_2$ or carbon dioxide is a gas which is naturally produced during respiration. The gas in itself is acidotic and as such it can dramatically affect the pH and acid-base balance of the patient. Carbon dioxide also has vasodilatory properties, which are important in caring for certain subgroups of patients for example head injured patients[8]. A normal PaCO$_2$ level is between 35 and 45 mmHg or 4.7 - 6.0 KPa[9]. Carbon dioxide is an indicator that an acidosis or alkalosis may be occurring due to a primary respiratory problem.

Base Excess

The base access is a figure which represents the amount of acid which is dissolved in the blood. Normal figures for a base excess is somewhere around -2 - +2[10]. A reading of -3 would indicate that there is more acid in the blood than is normal (strictly speaking a base excess of 0 would be normal) and a base excess of +3 would indicate that there is not enough acid in the blood. When the patient's base excess is deranged it is suggestive of a metabolic cause for the academia or alkalosis, unless there is a compensatory mechanism occurring (this will be discussed later).

Sodium bicarbonate

Sodium bicarbonate (or SBC) is produced by the kidneys amongst other organs. It is one of the main buffers or alkalising agents within the blood. If the bicarbonate level is too low then the patient is likely to become acidotic unless they have other compensatory mechanisms. Inversely if the bicarbonate is too high then the patient will likely become alkalotic. Acute renal failure will cause a drop in sodium bicarbonate being produced and subsequently an acidaemia will occur until other mechanisms start to compensate the situation. A normal sodium bicarbonate level with the 21 to 28 mmol per litre[3].

Haemoglobin

Haemoglobin is the oxygen carrying component of red blood cells, as such if there is not enough haemoglobin in the blood it is unlikely that the patient will have a satisfactory PaO_2. The patient may be displaying adequate or normal oxygen saturations, as the haemoglobin that is there is fully saturated with the oxygen, however there is not enough haemoglobin to produce a satisfactory PaO_2. Haemoglobin is also a buffer or alkalising agent. A normal haemoglobin level will be dependent on the age of the patient, but in the critically ill adult it is generally accepted that a haemoglobin level of less than 80 grams per litre would be an indicator to provide a blood transfusion[11].

Lactate

Lactate is an acid that is produced during anaerobic respiration. An inadequate supply of oxygen to the cell will cause an increase in lactate production and excretion. Lactate is therefore a good indicator of the cells demand versus supply of oxygen. It goes hand-in-hand that if there is poor perfusion then there will be poor oxygen delivery, despite the increased oxygen demand at the cellular level. Subsequently the lactate will rise occur as the cells begin anaerobic respiration. The increase in lactate production may not be detected until perfusion is rectified. A normal lactate is considered by some to be between 0.3 and 1.3 in the healthy not critically unwell patient, however less than 2 mmol per litre is accepted by many in the critical care setting[12].

Glucose

Glucose is simply that - the amount of glucose in the blood. Be aware that during a stress response of critical illness the glucose levels will be transiently raised until the stress response has been normalised[13]. A normal glucose level in the blood is between 4.4 and 6.1 mmols/L, or 82 to 110 mg/dL when fasting, or around 8mmols/L (144mg/dl) after eating. The exact figures are flexible, as the American Diabetes Association suggests that the blood glucose level should be kept below 10 mmols/L (180 mg/dL) and a fasting blood glucose should be kept between 5 to 7.2 mmols/L (90–130 mg/dL).[14, 15]

People with diabetes are more likely to have raised blood glucose levels and may need treatment with intravenous insulin during a critical illness to maintain glucose control. Equally patients with a critical illness are more likely to be exhibiting a stress response and will have higher glucose levels than normal, which will need monitoring and potential treatment.

The oxygen dissociation curve

The oxygen dissociation curve (ODC) is a somewhat challenging concept to comprehend. The following image explains the ODC.

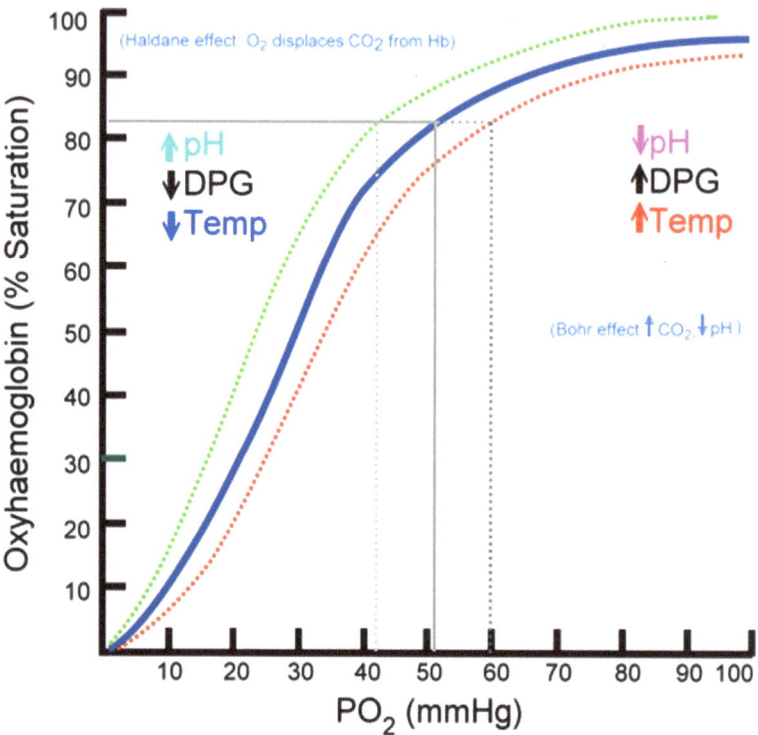

The previous image can be explained as follows: the dark blue, solid line depicts a normal pH, normal 2–3 DPG (2-3-diphosphoglycerate) and normal temperature; the dotted green line, above the solid blue line depicts a blood gas with an increase in pH, or a decrease in 2–3 DPG or a patient who is hypothermic; the dotted red line, below the solid blue line is an arterial blood gas with a decrease in pH, or an increase in 2–3 DPG or a patient who is hyperthermic. A patient who is alkalotic, or hypothermic will have a lower PaO_2 to achieve the same oxygen saturations as a normal pH or normal 2-3 DPG. Inversely, a patient who is hyperthermic, or is acidotic will need a higher PaO_2 to achieve the same oxygen saturations.

It is also important to note that the oxygen saturations drop considerably when the PaO_2 falls below is around 55mm Hg. The fall in PaO_2 and oxygen saturations are not uniformed, but instead follows a sigmoid shape, which means that at a certain point the oxygen saturations will fall rapidly.

2–3 DPG, which is also known by many names such as 2-3-diphosphoglycerate, 2-3 Bisphosphoglyceric acid, 2-3-Bisphosphoglycerate or 2,3-BPG. It is a substance that bonds to deoxygenated haemoglobin when there is a lower partial pressure of oxygen in the atmosphere[16]. It actually lowers the affinity of oxygen to haemoglobin, but inversely increases oxygens release at the cellular level[16]. An example of this is seen at altitude when an increase in the substance allows the person to have some improvement in their tissue oxygenation, as without it tissue hypoxia would be likely.

Temperature Correction

Many people wonder if temperature correction should be used for arterial blood gas interpretation. The quick answer is no. The reasons for this are as follows:

1. Entering the temperature correction values affects the values given on the PaO_2 and this may result in a higher PaO_2 being recorded. As mentioned a shift to the right or left will affect the affinity of oxygen to the heamoglobin, however it will inversely affect the release at the cellular level. As such a higher PaO_2 may make the user think that the patient is hyperoxygenated, however at the cellular level the tissues will not be getting as much oxygen. So if the user observes a higher PaO_2 they would tend to reduce to FiO_2 or other variable to bring the PaO_2 into a more acceptable range, which would further decrease the already potentially impaired oxygen delivery and supply to the tissues[5]. Also, if the PaO_2 was showing high on an arterial blood gas using the temperature correction model the user may increase the respiratory rate or pressures / volumes on a ventilator which may increase the patients risk of developing barotrauma or respiratory muscle weakness;

2. The main discussion in the literature currently relies on animal models to assess differences and reliability of temperature correction versus non-temperature correction. Until more human models support using temperature correction using this method of interpreting blood gasses should be avoided. This concept is widely accepted by many authority bodies[5].

3. There is a difference in the physiological association that the body has at varying temperatures which can further confuse the clinician if they use temperature correction[5]. An example of this is during hyperthermia the body has an increase in metabolic demand;

4. The alpha-stat method of arterial blood gas interpretation is the method of choice outside of cardiopulmonary bypass and post cardiac arrest where severe cooling is employed to protect the brain and reduce metabolic demand[5]. Alpha-stat is measuring the blood gas at 37°C.

Temperature correction is often used during cardiopulmonary bypass, however these patients are cooled to around 31°C and the results there are valid, however in the presence of a mild hypothermia greater than approximately 35°C and less than 40°C no temperature correction is needed[5]. One of the basic principles, however, is to ensure that whatever process is being used in the care facility, the process needs to be consistent. There is no point someone using temperature correction and the other clinician not using it, as inconsistencies will be present which will not directly represent the patient and their acid base or respiratory variables[5].

Arterial Blood Gas Interpretation and Analysis

Once the ABG has been taken it needs to be interpreted to understand what is occurring with the patient and to provide prompts for treatment options.

These are the steps that I advocate to interpret an ABG

1. Is the pH acidotic or alkalotic?

2. Is the $PaCO_2$ high or low?

3. Is the PaO_2 high or low?

4. Is the base excess within normal limits?

5. Is the sodium bicarbonate level normal?

6. Is the lactate normal?

7. Does the patient have a normal Hb?

8. Is the glucose level within normal limits?

In the next few sections I will give some varying examples of ABG's and their interpretation with suggestions on the treatments necessary. I will not make reference to steps 7 & 8, as simply if there is not enough Hb in the blood the oxygen carrying capacity will be significantly diminished and the patient's PaO_2 may be low. If this is the case a blood transfusion may be indicated and it may also be worth looking for any active bleeding to explain the low Hb level[11]. The glucose figure is important in the complete patient analysis, but it does not require in-depth analysis with regard to ABG interpretation: if the glucose level is high, insulin may be indicated; if it is low then more glucose may be warranted.

Carbon dioxide levels will change very rapidly to cause a shift in the patient's pH, however the patients base excess, lactate and sodium bicarbonate levels will take longer to alter. As such these metabolic changes will take longer for the affects to alter the patients' pH level[17].

Respiratory Acidosis

A respiratory acidosis is shown on an ABG as:

- pH less than 7.35

- $PaCO_2$ higher than 45mmHg or 6KPa

- Base Excess will be normal

- Lactate will be normal

- Sodium bicarbonate will be normal

  - pH = 7.2

  - $PaCO_2$ = 55mmHg

  - PaO_2 = 75mmHg

  - BE = +1.5

  - Sodium bicarbonate = 28 mmol/L

  - Lactate = 0.5

  - Hb = 110 g/L

With this example of a respiratory acidosis we can see that the patient is acidotic, by a raised carbon dioxide level and a normal base excess. It is interesting to see that the base excess is slightly elevated above the zero point and the sodium bicarbonate is at the upper limit of normal, which may indicate that the problem causing the respiratory acidosis has not "just" occurred, but may have started an hour ago or slightly more.

This presentation of a respiratory acidosis is often seen during an episode of acute hypoventilation.

Respiratory alkalosis

A respiratory alkalosis is presented as follows:

- A pH level of greater the 7.45

- A $PaCO_2$ of less than 35mmHg or 4.7KPa

- A normal base excess

- A normal lactate

- A normal sodium bicarbonate level

  - pH = 7.6

  - $PaCO_2$ = 30mmHg

  - PaO_2 = 95mmHg

  - BE = -0.9

  - Sodium bicarbonate = 21 mmol/L

  - Lactate = 0.9

  - Hb = 120 g/L

This example of a respiratory alkalosis clearly shows a higher than normal pH, with a low $PaCO_2$ and a normal base excess, sodium bicarbonate and lactate. Again the sodium bicarbonate level is on the lower side of normal, but it is still within normal limits - again suggesting that this may have been occurring for at least an hour[17].

The presentation of a respiratory alkalosis is often seen with hyperventilation[18].

Metabolic acidosis

A metabolic acidosis is common for a wide set of acutely unwell patients. They present with:

- A low pH (less than 7.35)

- A $PaCO_2$ which is normal

- A base excess which is more negative than -2

- With:

- A lactate which will be raised greater than 2 mmol/L, and/or

- A sodium bicarbonate level which will be lower than 21 mmol/L, and/or

- An Hb level which will be lower than 80.

The patient may display with a mixture of significant alteration of their lactate, sodium bicarbonate and haemoglobin, depending on the underlying cause for the metabolic acidosis. The main point, however, is that the $PaCO_2$ will be normal in the presence of an acidosis - excluding respiratory involvement.

- pH = 7.1

- $PaCO_2$ = 36 mmHg

- PaO_2 = 90 mmHg

- BE = -8

- Sodium bicarbonate = 22 mmols/L

- Lactate = 9

- Hb = 90 g/L

In this example of a metabolic acidosis we note that the pH is low with a normal $PaCO_2$ (although it is towards the lower end of the normal limits). The base excess is very low, which is matched with the very negative lactate and a sodium bicarbonate towards the lower end of the acceptable limits.

This is likely due to a hypo-perfused state, as the Hb is not too severe and the sodium bicarbonate is still considered within normal limits. This patient had a B/P of 60/40 due to septic shock, which he had been compensating haemodynamically for the last couple of days, but has acutely developed shock.

Metabolic alkalosis

A metabolic alkalosis is defined as follows:

- A pH higher than 7.45

- A $PaCO_2$ within normal limits

- A base excess of greater than +2

- A sodium bicarbonate level of greater than 28 mmols/L

- A normal lactate level

- The Hb level may be raised or normal

An example of this would be as follows:

- pH = 7.6

- $PaCO_2$ = 40

- PaO_2 = 90

- BE = +6

- Lactate = 0.5

- Sodium bicarbonate = 34

- Hb = 110

The previous example shows the high pH, with a normal CO_2 level. The BE is expected to be high in this case, due to the increased sodium bicarbonate present in the blood. The haemoglobin is within acceptable limits.

The causes of metabolic alkalosis are more challenging for the clinician, as the pH can be corrected more easily with a ventilated patient, however this does not fix the underlying problem causing the metabolic alkalosis.

Causes for each of the acidotic and alkalotic examples will be given later.

Compensation Of ABG's

The body, as mentioned previously, operates within a very tight pH level and as such it must attempt to compensate for any deviations in the actual pH of the blood to achieve a normal range, this is done a few ways. For a metabolic primary problem, the $PaCO_2$ will alter by either hyperventilation (tachypnoea or increased tidal volumes, which is the volume of gas inspired and subsequently expired on each breath) or hypoventilation (low respiratory rate and a lower tidal volume). With a primary respiratory deviation in the blood's pH the metabolic buffers will try to compensate for the pH change. Metabolic buffers include sodium bicarbonate, haemoglobin, phosphate, plasma proteins, ammonia and calcium carbonate[19]. Sodium bicarbonate is the main buffer used for alterations in blood pH to achieve normality, however haemoglobin is also important as it can attract carbon dioxide during increase cellular respiration[19]. Plasma proteins and phosphate play lesser roles as their concentrations are too low to achieve a significant change[19]. Calcium carbonate, which is found in bone is only useful during prolonged acidotic episodes[19].

Primary metabolic deviations in the patients' pH can be adjusted by the respiratory system rapidly, however primary respiratory deviations in the patients' pH are corrected by the metabolic buffers a lot slower and will take hours to compensate fully[17], as shown next.

Primary Respiratory Alkalosis

	Onset of acuity	2 hours	4 hours
pH	7.6	7.5	7.4

	Onset of acuity	2 hours	4 hours
PaCO2	25	25	25
PaO2	85	85	85
Base Excess	0	-3	-5.5
Sodium Bicarbonate	25	20	16
Lactate	0.5	0.5	0.5
Hb	97	97	97

Primary Respiratory Acidosis

	Onset of acuity	2 hours	4 hours
pH	7.2	7.3	7.4
PaCO2	60	60	60
PaO2	90	90	90
Base Excess	0	+3	+5.5

	Onset of acuity	2 hours	4 hours
Sodium Bicarbonate	25	30	35
Lactate	0.5	0.5	0.5
Hb	97	97	98

Primary Metabolic Alkalosis

	Onset of acuity	30 minutes	1 hour
pH	7.6	7.5	7.4
PaCO2	40	50	55
PaO2	90	95	100
Base Excess	+5.5	+5.5	+5.5
Sodium Bicarbonate	30	30	30
Lactate	0.5	0.5	0.5
Hb	97	97	98

Primary Metabolic Acidosis

	Onset of acuity	30 minutes	1 hour
pH	7.2	7.3	7.4
PaCO2	40	30	28
PaO2	90	85	80
Base Excess	-5.5	-5.5	-5.5
Sodium Bicarbonate	17	17	17
Lactate	0.5	0.5	0.5
Hb	97	97	97

Please note that the times are rough guides only and are not always going to be accurate. The times are just supposed to indicate that longer time is needed for compensation of primary respiratory issues.

Treatment Options Following Interpretation Of The Arterial Blood Gas

ABG's are often taken during critical illness by critical care professionals who love to "play" with numbers. It is fairly easy to manipulate ABG values to achieve normal values, however often the adjuncts that are needed to achieve the changes are just that - adjuncts; they do not fix the underlying problem that is causing the derangement. The primary focus needs to be on treating the underlying cause for the abnormalities in the ABG. An example of this would be a patient with hypoxaemia secondarily to a community acquired pneumonia. The clinician will give oxygen, which will often correct the abnormal blood gas values, but without the correct antibiotics the problem will not be correctly treated and the pneumonia is likely to worsen.

The patient in a non-critical care environment

The advanced treatment of an ABG is limited if the patient was outside of a critical care environment. More critical derangements in the ABG values obtained from the patient accompanied by a corresponding clinical assessment may negate that the patient needs to be accommodated within a critical care environment.

Hypoxaemia

There are five main reasons for hypoxaemia and they are:

1. Hypoventilation[20], caused by:

    1. Obesity;

    2. Decreased level of consciousness;

3. Muscular fatigue, such as muscular dystrophy or myasthenia gravis;

4. Neuromuscular disease such as Guillain-Barré disease or a high spinal injury;

5. Trauma such as a flail chest.

2. Diffusion reduction in the alveoli[20]:

1. Caused by interstitial lung disease or other substances that reduce the transport of oxygen through the alveoli.

3. Ventilation - Perfusion (VQ) mismatch[20]:

1. Pulmonary vascular disease, such as pulmonary embolism, pulmonary hypertension, pulmonary oedema;

2. Interstitial lung disease, or diffuse parenchymal lung disease which often result in pulmonary fibrosis after prolonged exposure. This can be caused by several substances for example asbestosis, chemotherapeutic medications, rheumatoid arthritis, systemic lupus erythematosus, tuberculosis, pneumocystis pneumonia, malignancies and many more.

4. Right to left shunt of the heart[20]:

1. Atrial and ventricular cardiac septal defects;

2. Pulmonary arteriovenous malformations;

3. Hepatopulmonary syndrome, which is increased arteriovenous dilation of the pulmonary micro circulation. This is seen in acute and chronic liver failure patients.

5. Reduced inspired oxygen content below 21%[20]:

1. Commonly seen at high altitude.

Hypoxaemia is treated by giving the patient enough oxygen to achieve a PaO_2 and SpO_2 within the patients normal range taking into account their present clinical condition. For example a patient with a pneumonia which is being treated in a ward environment may only realistically achieve a SpO_2 of 90%, which should correlate to a PaO_2 of around 80mmHg or 10.7 KPa. It would therefore be unrealistic to try to achieve a SpO_2 of 100% or a PaO_2 of greater than 100 or 13.3 KPa. Remember that a normal PaO_2 is greater than 83mmHg or 11.1KPa, so trying to achieve a higher value is often not necessary.

Other methods of increasing the V/Q mismatch need to be utilised, such as correct and adequate patient positioning, siting up as high as possible[21], ensuring analgesia is satisfactory to enable the patient to deep breath and cough and engaging in patient mobility wherever possible[22].

The patient may be anaemic and as such will not have enough oxygen carrying capacity to cause a normal PaO_2. A blood transfusion may be indicated.[11], as already discussed.

Treatment of the underlying condition needs to be attended to, whether it is antibiotics, frusemide, decreasing anti-sedative medications, mobility, deep breathing and coughing, anti-thrombolytics (although these are normally given in a critical care environment), bronchodilators, vasodilators - there are a multitude of treatments depending on the clinical condition.

An important point to note is that if the patient is known to be a chronic airways limitation (CAL) or chronic obstructive airways disease (COAD) sufferer they have a different mechanism to control their respiration. People not suffering from CAL or COAD control their respirations by a negative feedback loop related to the $PaCO_2$ controlled by chemoreceptors found in the carotids, aorta and in the medulla[23]. If their $PaCO_2$ level is high, then they hyperventilate by increasing their tidal volumes and their respiratory rate[23]. The person suffering with CAL or COAD, however, control their respirations from oxygen chemoreceptors. Therefore if the patient has a PaO_2 which is high, due to an excessive amount of oxygen being given to the patient they will hypoventilate, which will further increase their $PaCO_2$ and cause a reduced level of consciousness which will exacerbate their hypoventilation. In an acute, emergency situation, high amounts of oxygen can be given to COAD / CAL suffers[24], as patients do not arrest from hypercarbia (high CO_2 levels), they die from hypoxia[24]. It is important that after the high supplementary oxygen has been given that the patient is observed and they do not hypoventilate further.

A-a Gradient

The A-a gradient looks at the difference between the alveolar and arterial partial pressure of oxygen. The A-a gradient gives guidance with regard to the hypoxia being due to gas exchange difficulties which may be due to either:

- VQ mismatch, interstitial lung disease, or alveolar disease[25, 26]; or,

- Hypoventilation[25, 26]

It is important to know that the formula is only accurate at room air. It can be applied to higher FiO_2 situations, but the figure will not be accurate, but it should give guidance into the underlying issue with hypoxia.

The normal value is worked out as follows[25, 26]

$$(Age \times 0.21) + 2.5$$

So, for a 40 year old man a normal value would be:

$$(40 \times 0.21) + 2.5 = 10.9$$

To work out the value for the specific patient being assessed the following formula needs to be applied[25, 26]:

$$(FiO_2 \times (pAtm - pH_2O)) - (PaCO_2 / RespQuot) + (PaCO_2 \times FiO_2 \times (1- RespQout) / RespQuot) - PaO_2$$

pAtm = Atmospheric pressure, which at sea level is 760 mmHg[25, 26];

pH_2O = Water vapour pressure at 37°C = 47mmHg[25, 26];

RespQuot = Respiratory Quotient, which is a dimensionless number referring to the basal metabolic rate, which varies depending upon the type of food ingested. It is generally 0.8 in a "normal diet"[25, 26].

So, to work out the equation for our 40 year old man breathing room air, who has a PaO_2 of 91 and a $PaCO_2$ of 40 the equation is broken down as follows:

$$(0.21 \times (760 - 47)) - (40 / 0.8) + (40 \times 0.21 \times (1 - 0.8 / 0.8) - 91 = 10.83$$

If a patient has the same values, but a PaO_2 of 65 the results would be a figure of 36.83, which would be indicative of a gas exchange difficulties.

If a patient has a $PaCO_2$ of 55 and a PaO_2 of 73, the figure given would be 10.8675 which would greatly suggest hypoventilation as the figure is normal in the face of hypoxaemia.

With the previous example it is good to notice that although the PaO_2 is low and the $PaCO_2$ is high, by using the A-a gradient formula, hypoventilation is the probable cause of the hypoxaemia and not just hypoperfusion.

Hypercapnia

Hypercapnia is generally due to hypoventilation[27] and measures need to be taken to reverse the situation. Does the patient have a decreased level of consciousness which is causing them to hypoventilate, or does the patient have a significant pneumonia, or other lung pathology? Does the patient have a pneumothorax or haemothorax which needs treatment? Another common cause for hypoventilation is pain when deep breathing, so analgesia is an important factor to consider and ensuring it is being taken by the patient when indicated. Along with these clinical problems the patient may be suffering from acute pulmonary oedema, which may benefit from some frusemide.

Hypercapnia is often seen in the patient with CAL or COAD[28], so a permissive hypercapnia should be allowed in these patients,[29] however they should not be acidotic[30]. If they are, then that is an indicator that they are suffering an acute episode that needs treatment[30]. This is because COAD / CAL is a chronic condition, so the metabolic buffers have time to fully correct the pH in a "normal" setting. Therefore if the patient is acidotic or alkalotic then they are not compensating as they normally would do.

Another reason for hypercapnia is rebreathing exhaled CO_2[31].

If the patient is showing a high $PaCO_2$ and a high base excess then there is an element of compensation occurring and the primary cause for the either high $PaCO_2$ or a high base excess needs to be established. So, although the main reason for a high $PaCO_2$ is hypoventilation it is also possible to have a high $PaCO_2$ due to a metabolic alkalosis.

Acidaemia

Acid is formed in the body by the oxidation of amino acids, metabolism of glucose to form lactic acid and pyruvic acid but this is only a small amount of acid produced[32]. The majority of acid produced is due to CO_2 which is produced from aerobic respiration, which when added to water turns to carbonic acid, which then can then produce bicarbonate and a hydrogen (acid) ion. The equation is as follows[32]:

$$CO_2 + H_2O <=> H_2CO_3 <=> HCO_3^- + H^+$$

Respiratory acidaemia is caused by hypercapnia, so refer back to the previous section.

Metabolic acidosis is generally caused by either / or[32]:

1. Decrease in bicarbonate:

   1. Diarrhoea;

   2. Proximal renal tubule acidosis (type 2), which is due to the inability of the proximal tubule to reabsorb bicarbonate.

2. Increase in acid production:

   1. Lactic acidosis;

   2. Ketosis, which can be due to alcohol, uncontrolled diabetes, or starvation;

   3. Ingestion of ethylene glycol or methanol, which is found in antifreeze, windshield wiper fluid, cleaning products and other solvents.

3. Reduction in acid being excreted by the kidneys:

   1. Renal failure;

   2. Distal renal tubule acidosis (type 1), as the distal tubule is responsible for secreting acid and if it fails then acidaemia will occur.

The underlying cause for the acidaemia needs to be established. If the patient has an acidaemia due to a metabolic reason other more complex assessments need to be made. What is the patient's renal function and therefore their sodium bicarbonate level? If their renal function is not within normal limits their bicarbonate level should be lower. How is their fluid status, are they intravascularly hypovolaemic? Are they struggling to perfuse their tissues which is indicated by a raised lactate? This may be resolved in the ward environment by the administration of fluids and ensuring the blood pressure is adequate for the patient. Reduction or omission of medications that cause a decrease in the blood pressure may also be indicated.

Alkalosis

A respiratory alkalosis is caused hyperventilation, where an excessive amount of CO_2 is expired, causing a rise in pH (as CO_2 is an acid). Acute management of hyperventilation is by giving the patient reassurance and trying to get them to breath slower and deeper. If this is unsuccessful then a small dose of benzodiazepine may be indicated.

Metabolic alkalosis, however, has a few more causes, for example[33]:

1. A loss of hydrochloric acid, by excessive vomiting;

2. Dehydration:

   1. Including extravagant dieresis due to diuretics;

   2. Cushing's syndrome.

3. Consumption of alkaline substances.

Treatment for nausea mainly includes anti-emetics or prokinetics. Dehydration is treated by re-hydration, whilst paying close attention to the various electrolyte levels. Cushing's syndrome is usually due to a tumour and the treatments will vary depending upon the type and location;

however treatment includes surgery, radiotherapy and chemotherapy. Consumption of alkaline substances needs to be supported by treating the symptoms and presenting problems.

As with hypercapnia, if the patient has a high base excess for a period of time, the lungs will try to compensate for the rise in pH, by actively hypoventilating to raise the $PaCO_2$ and balance the pH.

The Patient In A Critical Care Environment

The treatment for a patient in a critical care environment is possibly a bit easier than a patient out of this clinical area, simply because of the adjuncts that are available to treat the imbalances.

All the treatments remain the same, as with the patient out of the critical care environment, however below is some additional critical care options.

Hypoxia

Hypoxia can be treated by using several devices:

1. Hi-Flow: This device flows oxygen, or an oxygen / air mix into the patient's nostrils at 30 - 50 litres per minute. This often reduces the work of breathing and increases the PaO_2 by giving a very small amount of PEEP (Positive End Expiratory Pressure). The amount of PEEP that these devices deliver depend upon the flow rates used, but range from approximately 2 - 4 cmH20 pressure;

2. CPAP (Continuous Positive Airways Pressure): This is a device which often is used by strapping a mask to the patients' face, ensuring it is air tight. Other ways of delivering CPAP include a hood over the patient's head, or for the very compliant patient a nose mask, which will only work if the patient keeps their mouth closed. This

device is based on the principle that if PEEP, which is often in the range of 5 - 10 and sometimes even up to 20 cmH_2O pressure, is applied to the airways and subsequently to the lungs and alveoli then they are likely to recruit collapsed alveoli sacs and splint smaller airways open. This process will aid oxygen transportation through the alveoli capillaries, increasing the patient's PaO_2. This is why CPAP is often used in pulmonary oedema, as the fluid can be pushed into the capillary vasculature and then excreted by the kidneys with the help of frusemide.

3. Invasive ventilation: This is common place in the intensive care unit (ICU). As such the methods for treating hypoxia also include:

    1. Endotracheal tube (ETT) suctioning;

    2. Increasing the tidal volumes, either by increasing the inspiratory pressures or the mandatory tidal volume (TV) on the ventilator to achieve 6 - 8mls/Kg of the patient's ideal body weight (IBW). It is true that increasing the patient's tidal volume has more of an impact on the CO_2 (to be discussed later), however a low TV will cause hypoxia also, however the hypercapnia should be more pronounced;

    3. If the patient is expiring fully, which can be observed by looking at the volume and flow curve, which should come back to the baseline, an option may be to increase the inspiratory time, because it is within this area of breathing that oxygen is transferred into the capillaries. Observation needs to be performed to ensure that the patient does not start "breath stacking", which is when not all the expired breath manages to leave the patient before another breath starts;

    4. Increasing PEEP is an option, however this may have some adverse effects ono the cardiovascular

system by increasing the resting intra-thoracic pressures and subsequently constricting the vasculature and heart. Also by increasing the PEEP, if the underlying volumes or pressures above the PEEP being delivered to the patient are not adjusted the peak airways pressures will increase and barotrauma may be the result, which is a concern. If PEEP is increased, then the volumes or pressures provided above the PEEP may need to be reduced to achieve the same peak airway pressure as was being received before the increase in PEEP;

5. Recruitment manoeuvres can be done, by slowly increasing either the PEEP, or the inspiratory pressure for a period of time and then dropping it back down to an optimum level after some time. Another method of recruitment is to provide and inspiratory hold for around 30 seconds. These methods are thought to open up collapsed areas of alveoli;

6. Varying the modes of ventilation:

1. Pressure Support Ventilation (PSV) or Assisted Spontaneous Breathing (ASB) is a mode that allows the patient to trigger all breaths, but when the patient inspires the ventilator provides some "pressure support" or "assistance" to compensate for the increased work of breathing or resistance of the ETT which the patient needs to overcome to breath through. The patient cannot hold their breath on this mode of ventilation, as the expiratory valve opens when the flow decreases by a set amount. It is the least aggressive mode of invasive ventilation, therefore if the patient is hypoxic on this mode and all measures have been exhausted and the patient is getting beyond a fractional index of inspired oxygen (FiO_2) of 0.5 - 0.6 (which is the same as

50% or 60% oxygen), then the patient may need to move onto either a volume controlled or pressure controlled mode of ventilation;

2. Synchronised Intermittent Mandatory Ventilation with PSV or ASB (SIMV), is a mode of ventilation which will provide a minimum set rate of breathing per minute and when the patient decides he / she wants to trigger a spontaneous breath they can with the help of the PSV or ASB. This mode is conventionally known as a volume controlled mode which provides a set TV for each of the mandatory breaths over a set inspiratory time (Tinsp), however some ventilators also have SIMV with a pressure control mode, which will deliver a set respiratory rate (RR) at a set pressure above the PEEP over a set Tinsp. The patient will receive as much of the TV as is possible until they reach the set pressure (Pinsp) on the ventilator. If the patient is hypoxic on the PSV or ASB mode alone, then the SIMV with PSV/ASB mode would be an appropriate escalation. Should this mode not be suitable for the patient then they may have to escalate to the next mode;

3. Pressure Control Ventilation (PCV), which is sometimes called Pressure Control Ventilation Assist (PCV+A). This is the most aggressive form of conventional ventilation which will deliver as much TV as is possible to achieve the Pinsp above the PEEP over a set Tinsp. This is the same as SIMV with PSV / ASB in the pressure control setting, however what is different is that when the patient decides to take a spontaneous breath above the set rate they receive the same Tinsp as the mandatory breaths. This is in opposition to the expiratory valve opening when the flow decreases a certain amount. In this

mode the patient cannot expire until the Tinsp has been completed. This can be a very uncomfortable mode of ventilation for the patient and as such good levels of sedation may be necessary. Should this mode of ventilation not be correcting the respiratory response then consultation should be made with a tertiary service who can offer advice and potentially offer some more advanced forms of ventilation or oxygenation therapies.

4. Hi-Frequency Oscillating Ventilation (HFOV) is a type of ventilation which keeps the airways continuously open at a higher mean airway pressure than conventional ventilation. The patient will receive around 500 breaths per minute. This mode is often used for a severe respiratory acidosis which has not responded to conventional therapies and as such it is generally used in hypercapnic situations, however the patient may be hypoxic. To help you, the reader, I have included all modes of ventilation / oxygenation here together.

5. Extra Corporeal Membrane Oxygenation (ECMO) is used when all other modes of ventilation have failed. This is a very advanced and technically challenging form of oxygenating the blood by taking the blood from the patient and passing it through an oxygenator and putting it back into the patient. It is only performed by specialised tertiary referral centres. It has some similarities to a cardio-pulmonary bypass machine.

Hypercapnia

Again, all the treatment options remain the same as with the patient out of the critical care environment, however there are some additional methods of correcting a raised CO_2 which can only be performed in a critical care area as follows:

1. Hi-Flow ventilation will make a very small amount of change to the $PaCO_2$, however it is probably not clinically significant, so this mode should only be used if the patient is not going to tolerate BiPAP (discussed next) and the patient is not for intubation;

2. In the conscious patient, if their $PaCO_2$ is raised due to ineffective respiration accompanied by an increased work of breathing Biphasic, or Bi-Level, Positive Airway Pressure (BiPAP) may be indicated. It is the same as CPAP, where a PEEP is set, however in this mode of non-invasive ventilation the Pinsp is set so the patient will get a satisfactory TV. In some of the BiPAP machines the patient does not receive a mandatory Tinsp until their RR falls below a set level. The clinician needs to be aware of this issue and the effects it may have on oxygenation and CO_2 exhalation. Careful attention needs to be made to the time left for expiration after the Tinsp prior the next breath starting. Should this mode of non-invasive ventilation be ineffective for the patient further invasive modes of ventilation may be necessary;

3. Invasive ventilation in either SIMV with PSV / ASB or PCV+A may be necessary. The PSV mode alone is probably not appropriate, as when the patient is having BiPAP they are essentially having a non-invasive form of PSV, so if they fail on BiPAP then they should not tolerate PSV ventilation immediately. Sedation will make a difference and relax the patient, however PSV should be reserved for when the patient is out of an acute phase and getting ready for extubation. With the intubated patient who is hypercapnic there are several ventilator associated options available including:

1. Aiming for a TV of 6 - 8 mls/kg which can be achieved by either increasing the set TV directly when in a volume controlled mode, or increasing the Pinsp to achieve an adequate TV when in a pressure controlled mode of ventilation. Be aware that caution needs to be made when increasing the peak airway pressures above 30cmH$_2$O. Peak airway pressure is the pressure of PEEP + Pinsp;

2. Increasing the RR will increase the minute volume (MV) and as such should decrease the PaCO$_2$, unless the patient is unable to expire all of their gasses, in which case "breath stacking" may occur;

3. Ensure that the patient is not "breath stacking"; if they are, then disconnecting them from the ventilator to allow for the additional non-expired gas to escape. When that is done either decrease the Tinsp or the RR to allow for longer expiratory time (Texp).

Acidosis

Again, the same principles apply to the patient in a critical care environment as they do to a patient in a non-critical care environment, however additional therapies can be offered in these higher level care areas.

Respiratory acidosis is caused by hypercapnia, so refer back to the previous section.

Metabolic acidosis in the critical care population can be due to several reasons, including the broad examples given previously. Other examples would include:

1. Sepsis[34];

2. Cardiac failure[35];

3. Metformin toxicity[36];

4. Malignancy[37];

5. HIV[38];

6. Alcoholism[39];

7. Following a jejunal bypass or other small bowel resections[40];

8. Fasting[41];

9. Asprin and salicylate overdose[42]; and,

10. Toluene or "glue-sniffing" inhalation overdose[43].

Treatment varies depending upon the underlying cause. Sepsis will be treated with intravenous antibiotics. Vasopressors, ventilation and renal replacement therapy may also be indicated.

Cardiac failure in the acute phase with a metabolic acidosis is treated by the introduction of inotropes to improve contractility and reduce after-load. Vasopressors, however may also be necessary in the hypotensive patient. In severe cardiac failure the use of an intra-aortic balloon pump may be indicated, or the use of veno-arterial ECMO. Some tertiary hospitals offer right ventricular assist device (RVAC), left ventricular assist devices (LVAD), or bi-ventricular assist device (BiVAD). These ventricular assist devices are often used as a bridge to heart transplantation.

Metformin toxicity in the very acute stage following ingestion may warrant activated charcoal. Fluids are used to treat hypotension, vasopressors may be needed in severe cases. There is controversy regarding the use of sodium bicarbonate infusions to correct the metabolic acidosis[44], however in the severe cases where the pH is <7.1 continuous renal replacement therapy (CRRT) is often required.

Malignancies are treated according to the type of malignancy, however treatment options include radiotherapy, chemotherapy and surgery.

Patients suffering from HIV can get a metabolic acidosis for any of the reasons stated previously, however they can also get a metabolic acidosis due to their anti-retrovirals - namely the nucleoside reverse transcriptase inhibitors (NRTI), which cause the mitochondria to become toxic causing a decrease in the energy production and an increase in lactate[45]. The treatment is often to stop the NRTI and find an alternative once the acidosis has resolved[46].

Metabolic acidosis due to alcoholism is treated with fluids, thiamine[47] and in some cases phosphates are needed to correct any deficit[48].

Jejunal bypass and small bowel resections can increase the patients risk of suffering from D-lactic acidosis, which is where glucose is ingested and not fully absorbed which increases the risk of production of d-lactate secondary to bacteria[49]. Treatment is intravenous antibiotics and sodium bicarbonate administration[49], which as already mentioned is controversial.

Fasting induced metabolic acidosis is treated with glucose and saline rehydration[47].

Aspirin or salicylate overdose is often treated with fluid resuscitation whilst being cautious of the non-cardiogenic pulmonary oedema that tends to present more commonly with the older population who are chronically toxic[50]. Vasopressors may be necessary in the correction of the hypotension. Activated charcoal is also often given, with intravenous glucose due to cerebral glucose levels being low, despite a normal blood glucose level[51]. Sodium bicarbonate administration is provided to neutralise the metabolic acidosis, whilst ensuring that hypokalaemia is corrected[52]. CRRT is also offered in the severe salicylate overdose.

Toluene or "glue sniffing", which is usually carried out by young persons who are usually unaware of the potential risk of a metabolic acidosis and what may follow. Toluene is found in marker pens, paints, enamels, lacquers and paint thinners. Treatment for toluene induced metabolic acidosis is supportive. Assessing the airway and breathing for decreased ventilation and increased risk of aspiration and intubating if this is a concern. Circulatory shock needs to be treated if present in the usual manner of fluids and if that does not raise the blood pressure vasopressors may be necessary. Psychiatric and psychosocial care is needed post the acute phase.

Alkalosis

A respiratory alkalosis is due to hyperventilation, which has been discussed previously. Reference should be made to that section in this book.

A metabolic alkalosis is due to the following:

1. Loss of gastrointestinal hydrogen:

    1. Vomiting;

    2. Adenoma or factitious diarrhoea due to laxative abuse (diarrhoea usually causes a metabolic acidosis, but in these two cases a metabolic alkalosis is the result)[53].

2. Loss of hydrogen from kidneys:

    1. Primary hyper-secretion of mineralocorticoids which include adrenal adenoma (Conn's syndrome), bilateral idiopathic adrenal hyperplasia, primary (unilateral) adrenal hyperplasia, aldosterone-producing adrenocortical carcinoma, familial hyperaldosteronism, glucocorticoid-remediable aldosteronism, familial hyperaldosteronism type II, ectopic aldosterone-producing adenoma or carcinoma[54];

    2. Diuretics;

3. Following correction of a respiratory acidosis where the pH is normalised. This causes the $PaCO_2$ to return to normal, however the bicarbonate remains at a high level in the blood for some time and subsequently a metabolic alkalosis remains until the bicarbonate level normalises;

4. Hypercalcaemia, which increases bicarbonate reabsorption. This is often seen in milk-alkali syndrome, where calcium carbonate is ingested, which causes renal failure. This then causes an increase in bicarbonate build-up and a reduction in bicarbonate excretion.

3. Intracellular shift of hydrogen:

1. Hypokalaemia, as when potassium is excreted it attracts hydrogen to be excreted also. In addition to this process, intracellular potassium leave the cells to go extracellular to replace the loss, however to achieve the correct electrical charge in the cell, hydrogen goes into the cells. This further exacerbates the metabolic alkalosis[55].

4. Administration of an alkali:

1. Should a large amount of bicarbonate be given it will obviously cause an alkalosis, however the renal system is very good as excreting bicarbonate, so unless renal failure is present the kidneys will try to overcome this[55];

2. Lactate and acetate is metabolised to bicarbonate by the liver, so if a large amount of lactate is given then an alkalosis may occur in the presence of renal failure[55];

3. Crack-cocaine use, which contains a large content of alkaline compounds, in patients suffering from renal failure will cause an alkalosis[55];

4. Fresh frozen plasma replacement fluid used in plasmapheresis[55].

5. Contraction of alkalosis:

1. When fluids free from bicarbonate are lost from the body, the concentration of bicarbonate in the body rises and a metabolic alkalosis occurs[56]. This is usually buffered however by the intracellular buffers[56];

2. Diuretics, used for the oedematous patient, helps to excrete bicarbonate free fluid from the patient. This is exacerbated by hydrogen loss.

The treatment of a metabolic alkalosis is a bit simpler than the causes. It is broken up into three principles:

1. Correct the volume deficit caused by vomiting, villious adenoma and diuretics. This reduces the amount of sodium that is retained in the body and subsequently therefore reducing the reabsorption of bicarbonate;

2. Replace potassium deficit. As previously mentioned hypokalaemia causes potassium to leave the cells and hydrogen enters the cells causing a metabolic alkalosis. If potassium is replaced this process is reversed;

3. Replacing chloride causes an increase in hydrogen secretion and correct the alkalosis.

Special considerations apply to the oedematous patient, for who sodium chloride fluid replacement would be inappropriate as it would make the oedema potentially worse. In these patients they are often hypokalaemic, so the administration of potassium chloride will correct the hypokalaemia and the metabolic alkalosis.

Acetazolamide is another option in the oedematous patient, as this drug reduces the reabsorption of sodium bicarbonate in the kidney and as such it will correct both the alkalosis and the hypervolaemia.

There are also some reports of hydrochloric acid being given when acetazolamide is not providing the desired effect[57].

Anion Gap

Assessing the anion gap (AG) is an important factor when assessing the causes for the patients metabolic acidosis. The acceptable anion gap varies between laboratories. Some places accepted 7 - 13 meq/L traditionally, however with newer laboratory analysers a range of 3 - 9 is seen as acceptable due to higher sodium chloride concentrations being measured[58].

The calculation is derived from sodium, chloride and bicarbonate. Some clinicians also add potassium to the equation, when this occurs the acceptable meq/L rises by approximately 4.

The varying equations are:

- Serum AG = Na- (Cl + HCO3)

- Serum AG = (Na + K) - (Cl + HCO3)

Be aware that in the presence of hypoalbuminaemia: for every 1 g/dL drop in albumin, the AG acceptable range will drop by 2.3 - 2.5 meq/L[59]. Equally in hyperalbuminaemia the acceptable range of the AG will rise in the same proportion and by the same ratio[59].

If there is a high AG then sources for the metabolic acidosis need to be found, however if the AG is within normal limits it is often due to hyperchloraemia.

Some clinicians prefer the use of "MUDPILES" as a prompt to remember the causes of the various metabolic acidosis:

- Methanol;
- Uremia;
- Diabetic ketoacidosis;
- Propylene glycol (deicer and antifreeze);
- Isoniazid (tuberculosis medication);
- Lactic acidosis;
- Ethylene glycol (antifreeze);
- Salicylates.

Bibliography

1. Doig, A.K., et al., Graphical arterial blood gas visualization tool supports rapid and accurate data interpretation. CIN: Computers, Informatics, Nursing, 2011. 29(4 (Suppl)): p. TC53-60.

2. Wikipedia. Arterial Blood Gas. 2012 10/10/2012]; Available from: http://en.wikipedia.org/wiki/Arterial_blood_gas.

3. Radiometer, The Blood Gas Handbook, 2011.

4. Rao, L.V. and M.J. Mitchell, Wallach's Interpretation of Diagnostic Tests. 9 ed2011: Lippincott Williams & Wilkins.

5. Bisson, J. and J. Younker, Correcting arterial blood gases for temperature: (when) is it clinically significant? Nursing in Critical Care, 2006. 11(5): p. 232-238.

6. Nogueira, P.M., et al., Central venous saturation: a prognostic tool in cardiac surgery patients. Journal of Intensive Care Medicine, 2010. 25(2): p. 111-116.

7. Christensen, M., Mixed venous oxygen saturation monitoring revisited: thoughts for critical care nursing practice. Australian Critical Care, 2012. 25(2): p. 78-90.

8. Paul, R.L., et al., Intracranial pressure responses to alterations in arterial carbon dioxide pressure in patients with head injuries. J Neurosurg, 1972. 36(6): p. 714-20.

9. Payne, S.J., et al., Effects of arterial blood gas levels on cerebral blood flow and oxygen transport. Biomedical Optics Express, 2011. 2(4): p. 966-979.

10. Fischbach, F.T. and M.B. Dunning, A Manual of Laboratory and Diagnostic Tests. 8 ed2009: Lippincott Williams & Wilkins.

11. Carson, J.L., et al., Red Blood Cell Transfusion: A Clinical Practice Guideline From the AABB. Annals of Internal Medicine, 2012. 157: p. 49-58.

12. Phypers, B. and J.M.T. Pierce, Lactate physiology in health and disease. Continuing Education in Anaesthesia, Critical Care & Pain, 2006. 6(3): p. 128-132.

13. Moitra, V.K. and B. Sweitzer, Preoperative Assessment and Management. 2 ed2008: Lippincott Williams & Wilkins.

14. Association, A.D., Standards of Medical Care in Diabetes. Diabetes Care, 2006. 29(Supplement 1): p. S4-S42.

15. Association, A.D., Screening for Type 2 Diabetes. CLINICAL DIABETES, 2000. 18(2).

16. Wikipedia. 2,3-Bisphosphoglyceric acid. 2012 [cited 2012 10/10/2012]; Available from: http://en.wikipedia.org/wiki/2,3-Bisphosphoglyceric_acid.

17. Pierce, N.F., D.S. Fedson, and K.L. Brigham, The Ventilatory Response to Acute Base Deficit in Humans. Time Course During Development and Correction of Metabolic Acidosis. Annals of Internal Medicine, 1970. 72: p. 633.

18. Madias, N.E., W.B. Schwartz, and J.J. Cohen, The maladaptive renal response to secondary hypocapnia during chronic HCl acidosis in the dog. Journal of Clininical Investigations 1977. 60: p. 1393.

19. Brandis, K. Acid-Base Physiology: Buffering. 2012 13/10/2012]; Available from: http://www.anaesthesiamcq.com/AcidBaseBook/ab2_2.php.

20. Williams, A.J., ABC of oxygen: assessing and interpreting arterial blood gases and acid-base balance. British Medical Journal, 1998. 317: p. 1213.

21. Tyson, S.F. and P. Nightingale, The effects of position on oxygen saturation in acute stroke: a systematic review. Clinical rehabilitation, 2004. 18(8): p. 863-871.

22. Siffleet, J., et al., Patients' self-report of procedural pain in the intensive care unit. Journal of Clinical Nursing, 2007. 16(11): p. 2142-2148.

23. Spector, N. and D. Klein, Chronic Critically Ill Dyspneic Patients: Mechanisms and Clinical Measurement. American Association of Critical Care Nurses, 2001. 12(2): p. 220-233.

24. Azeemuddin, A. and M.A. Graber. Evaluation of the adult with dyspnea in the emergency department. 2012 13/10/2012]; Available from: http://www.uptodate.com/contents/evaluation-of-the-adult-with-dyspnea-in-the-emergency-department?source=search_result&search=V%2FQ+mismatch&selectedTitle=6~67.

25. Kanber, G.J., F.W. King, and Y.R. Eshchar, The alveolar-arterial oxygen gradient in young and elderly men during air and oxygen breathing. The American Review of Respiratory Disease, 1968. 97(3): p. 376-381.

26. Mellemgaard, K., The alveolar-arterial oxygen difference: its size and components in normal man.

Acta Physiologica Scandinavica, 1966. 67(1): p. 10-20.

27. Schafer, T., [Method for measuring respiration in sleep: capnography for determining ventilation]. [German]. Biomedizinische Technik. Biomedical engineering, 2003. 48(6): p. 170-175.

28. Chan, C.S., et al., Eucapnia and hypercapnia in patients with chronic airflow limitation. The role of the upper airway. American Review of Respiratory Disease, 1990. 141(4 Part 1): p. 861-865.

29. Edrich, T. and N. Sadovnikoff, Anesthesia for patients with severe chronic obstructive pulmonary disease. . Current Opinion in Anaesthesiology, 2010. 23(1): p. 18-24.

30. Brander, P.E., [Noninvasive ventilation and acute respiratory failure]. [Review] [Finnish] Duodecim, 2011. 127(2): p. 167-175.

31. David, P., et al., Postural control and ventilatory drive during voluntary hyperventilation and carbon dioxide rebreathing. European Journal of Applied Physiology, 2012. 112(1): p. 145-154.

32. Post, T.W. and B.D. Rose. Approach to the adult with metabolic acidosis 2010 14/10/2012]; Available from: http://www.uptodate.com/contents/approach-to-the-adult-with-metabolic-acidosis?source=search_result&search=acidemia&selectedTitle=1~125.

33. Rose, B.D. Causes of metabolic alkalosis 2010 14/10/2010]; Available from: http://www.uptodate.com/contents/causes-of-metabolic-alkalosis?source=search_result&search=alkalosis&selectedTitle=1~150.

34. Gomella, L.G. and S.A. Haist. Laboratory Diagnosis: Chemistry, Immunology, Serology. 2007 15/10/2012]; 11:[Available from: http://proxy14.use.hcn.com.au/content.aspx?aID=26 99454.

35. Fulop, M., et al., Lactic acidosis in pulmonary edema due to left ventricular failure. Annals of Internal Medicine, 1973. 79: p. 180.

36. Gomella, L.G. and S.A. Haist. Commonly Used Medications. Clinician's Pocket Reference 2012 15/10/2010]; 11:[Available from: http://proxy14.use.hcn.com.au/content.aspx?aID=26 96124.

37. Sillos, E.M., J.L. Shenep, and G.A. Burghen, Lactic acidosis: a metabolic complication of hematologic malignancies: case report and review of the literature. Cancer, 2001(92): p. 2237.

38. John, M. and S. Mallal, Hyperlactatemia syndromes in people with HIV infection. Current Opinion in Infectious Disease, 2002. 15: p. 23.

39. Wrenn, K.D., et al., The syndrome of alcoholic ketoacidosis. Americal Journal of Medicine, 1991. 91: p. 119.

40. Bongaerts, G., J. Tolboom, and T. Naber, D-lactic acidemia and aciduria in pediatric and adult patients with short bowel syndrome. Clinical Chemistry, 1995. 41: p. 107.

41. Kitabchi, A.E. and B.D. Rose. Clinical features and diagnosis of diabetic ketoacidosis and hyperosmolar hyperglycemic state in adults. 2012 17/10/2012]; Available from: http://www.uptodate.com/contents/clinical-features-and-diagnosis-of-diabetic-ketoacidosis-and-

hyperosmolar-hyperglycemic-state-in-adults?source=see_link.

42. Gabow, P.A., et al., Acid-base disturbances in the salicylate-intoxicated adult. Archives of Internal Medicine, 1978. 138: p. 1481.

43. Streicher, H.Z., P.A. Gabow, and A.H. Moss, Syndromes of toluene sniffing in adults. Annals of Internal Medicine, 1981. 94: p. 758.

44. Teale, K.F., et al., The management of metformin overdose. Anaesthesia, 1998. 53: p. 698.

45. Brinkman, K. Mitochondrial toxicity of HIV nucleoside reverse transcriptase inhibitors. 2012 17/10/2012]; Available from: http://www.uptodate.com/contents/mitochondrial-toxicity-of-hiv-nucleoside-reverse-transcriptase-inhibitors?source=see_link&anchor=H12#H12.

46. Brinkman, K. Treatment and prevention of mitochondrial toxicity in HIV-infected patients. 2012 17/10/2012]; Available from: http://www.uptodate.com/contents/treatment-and-prevention-of-mitochondrial-toxicity-in-hiv-infected-patients?source=see_link.

47. Höjer, J., Severe metabolic acidosis in the alcoholic: differential diagnosis and management. Human & Experimental Toxicology, 1996. 15: p. 482.

48. Levy, L.J., et al., Ketoacidosis associated with alcoholism in nondiabetic subjects. Annals of Internal Medicine, 1973. 78: p. 213.

49. Halperin, M.L. and K.S. Kamel, D-lactic acidosis: turning sugar into acids in the gastrointestinal tract. Kidney International, 1996. 49: p. 1.

50. Chalasani, N., J. Roman, and R.L. Jurado, Systemic inflammatory response syndrome caused by chronic salicylate intoxication. Southern Medical Journal, 1996. 89: p. 479.

51. Kuzak, N., J.R. Brubacher, and J.R. Kennedy, Reversal of salicylate-induced euglycemic delirium with dextrose. Clinical Toxicology, 2007. 45: p. 526.

52. Proudfoot, A.T., E.P. Krenzelok, and J.A. Vale, Position Paper on urine alkalinization. Journal of Clinical Toxicology, 2004. 42: p. 1.

53. Perez , G.O., J.R. Oster, and A. Rogers, Acid-base disturbances in gastrointestinal disease. Digestive Diseases and Sciences, 1987. 32: p. 1033.

54. Williams textbook of endocrinology. 11th ed2008: Saunders/Elsevier.

55. Rose, B.D. and T.W. Post, Clinical Physiology of Acid-Base and Electrolyte Disorders. 5th ed2001: McGraw-Hill.

56. Garella, S., B.S. Chang, and S.I. Kahn, Dilution acidosis and contraction alkalosis: review of a concept. Kidney International, 1975. 8: p. 279.

57. Knutsen, O.H., New Method for Administration of Hydrochloric Acid in Metabolic Alkalosis. Lancet, 1983. 1: p. 953.

58. Winter, S.D., J.R. Pearson, and P.A. Gabow, The fall of the serum anion gaop. Archives of Internal Medicine, 1990. 150: p. 311.

59. Feldman, M., N. Soni, and B. Dickson, Influence of hypoalbuminaemia or hyperalbuminaemia on the serum anion gap. Journal of Laboratory and Clinical Medicine, 2005. 146: p. 317.

www.ingramcontent.com/pod-product-compliance
Lightning Source LLC
Chambersburg PA
CBHW041108180526
45172CB00001B/161